HAPPY OILS

Transform your beauty, health and
happiness with Aromatherapy

Faye Hurley

ISBN-13: 978-1499318746

SBN-10: 149931874X

DEDICATION

This book is dedicated to the people I love the most: my children and my fiancé. Sophie, Jasmine, Ethan, Isaac and Jason - you are at the heart of my wellbeing, and I love you more than words can say. I pray that you are blessed with a lifetime of happiness. It is also dedicated to the survivors of domestic abuse, who will gain the support they need, via the profits from this book. This book was written for you. Your 'value is far above rubies' and you deserve a life of happiness too.

CONTENTS

ACKNOWLEDGMENTS

Firstly, I want to thank God, who deserves far more honour than I can ever express; for giving me my passions, life purpose and the inspiration to write this book. I would like to thank my children and fiancé for putting up with my numerous nights spent tapping away on the computer over the last six months! I would like to thank my beautiful graphic designer, Lucy, for magically turning my scrawl into something which looks gorgeous. Finally, thank you to my family and friends for being my proof readers (whether they liked it or not!), and for their opinions and support.

1

INTRODUCTION

Essential oils are amazing!

They have long been known as 'Nature's Medicine Cabinet', with their ability to heal us physically, mentally and emotionally; and thereby increase our happiness.

Imagine that you are walking around a beautiful garden on a sunny day, and you can smell the gorgeous flower scents wafting through the air. Similarly, imagine walking into a florists that has an abundance of flowers and bouquets within it, which envelope you with their fragrance. How does this make you feel?

Does it lift your spirits, and make you smile as you're thinking about it now? Well that's what aromatherapy is ... it's using the beautiful essence of flowers, in a variety of ways, in order to help you to feel good!

Your sense of smell is so important - what we taste is dependent on it, our memories are connected to it, it can help us to feel energized or relaxed. Our sense of smell affects our mind, our emotions and our bodies - and yet we often take it for granted.

The aromas used in aromatherapy come from essential oils. They are the very 'essence' of the flower they came from; the fluids which cause the flower to have its fragrance.

Essential oils can be derived not only from petals, but also from herbs, seeds, leaves, stalks, wood bark, resin, fruit rind. A great example of this is the Bitter Orange Tree. You can obtain Petitgrain essential oil from its leaves and twigs, Neroli essential oil from its flowers as well as the Bitter Orange essential oil from the rind of its fruits. So that's three essential oils from only one tree!

There are thousands of essential oils, and each one can have a huge range of therapeutic benefits, such as being anti-inflammatory, energizing, sedative, uplifting, or even aphrodisiac!

Ultimately, once the essential oils have made their way into your body, they are your secret weapon for helping you to feel good, and this book has been written to show you how to use them in order for them do just that.

This book has been created with beginners in mind. Therefore, I have chosen to exclude any carrier oils and essential oils, which could potentially cause any adverse reactions or allergies (such as Sweet Almond Oil or Wheat germ Oil), and instead focus on a core group of oils which are generally considered to be the safest.

You will see that this easily manageable group can still heal a huge quantity of health ailments, and still provides you with a wealth of benefits for your wellbeing.

This book has been written to share the transformational joy that aromatherapy can bring, and I hope you love it as much as I do!

2

SAFETY WITH ESSENTIAL OILS

Most essential oils are very safe to use, however there are certain rules which must be followed. This book contains information on only a select few essential oils, which are generally considered to be some of the safest oils to use, but the following rules must still be adhered to:

- Do not use essential oils internally.
- Do not apply directly to skin; always dilute with carrier oil/base.
- Always do a 'Patch Test' to test for allergic reaction. Mix your Blend (in either a 1% or 2% dilution as appropriate) *(See notes on 'Your Rescue Kit & How to Create a Blend' to find out how to do this)*, and then apply the Blend onto the skin of the inner arm opposite the elbow (i.e.: the 'crook' of the arm).
  Do this preferably a couple of days prior to using the Blend. If any reaction/allergy occurs, discontinue use.
- Keep essential oils out of reach of children.
- Avoid contact with eyes and mucous membranes.

- Do not use citrus oils before exposure to UV light.

- Use only pure essential oils; avoid synthetic fragrances. Use essential oils of excellent quality, bought from reputable companies.

- **Do not use essential oils on babies, children (under the age of 11), pregnant women, the elderly, or those with serious/non serious health problems (asthma, epilepsy, cancer, diabetes, heart conditions, high/low blood pressure, varicose veins, fever, infectious diseases, osteoporosis) without advanced medical study. For the purposes of this book, I would advise that you <u>only</u> treat healthy (non pregnant) adults.**

- Always use essential oils in a well ventilated room. Prolonged exposure to essential oils without ventilation, can cause dizziness, nausea, light headedness, headaches, blood sugar imbalances and irritability.

- Store essential oils and carrier oils properly in a cool, dark room to avoid degradation and rancidity. Always keep your oils tightly sealed.

- Take special precautions with applications near delicate skin areas.

- **Do not massage, or use essential oils on broken skin, cuts, open wounds, fractures, recent surgery, inflammation/swelling etc.**

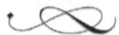

Before experimenting with an oil, become familiar with its properties, dose, and precautions. Many essential oils have contraindications (when in doubt about a condition or an oil, consult a qualified medical specialist/ aromatherapist). These are the contraindications of the essential oils specifically mentioned in this book:

Bergamot & Orange (or any citrus oils) should not be used before exposure to sunlight/sun beds.

Geranium should not be used on anyone who is Hypoglycaemic.

Jasmine & Peppermint can occasionally be a skin irritant to those with sensitive skin, so only use a low dosage.

The chemical groups for the essential oils mentioned in this book are:

Terpenes: Antiviral, Antiseptic, Anti-inflammatory.

Esters: Relaxing, Fungicidal.

Alcohols: Uplifting, Antiseptic, Antiviral.

3

YOUR RESCUE KIT &
HOW TO
CREATE A BLEND

This chapter describes the benefits of ten popular, and extremely versatile, essential oils. You can then select any number of these to create your personal home 'Rescue Kit'.

Choosing the essential oils which you feel are the most appropriate for you will create an easily manageable and personalised kit.

1. BERGAMOT
is joyful and uplifting

> Chemical group: *Ester & Alcohol*
> Price: *Inexpensive*
> Extraction: *Expression of the rind/peel*

BENEFITS:

- Can reduce symptoms of stress, depression, anxiety and fear.

- Can uplift and increase joyfulness, positivity, focus, confidence.

- Can ease symptoms of PMT, Cystitis, Varicose veins, Warts/Veruccas/Viral infections, Asthma and signs of ageing.

2. ROMAN CHAMOMILE OR GERMAN CHAMOMILE (AKA BLUE CHAMOMILE)
are calming

> Chemical group: *Ester & Terpene (Roman),*
> *Terpene & Alcohol (German)*
> Price: *Expensive*
> Extraction: *Steam distillation of the flowers*

BENEFITS:
- Can reduce symptoms of stress, depression, anxiety, anger, fear, rejection and grief.
- Can help you to relax and increase feelings of peace and contentment.
- Can ease symptoms of Menopause, PMT, Psoriasis/Eczema, Aches/Pains (inc. headaches, arthritis), Fertility/Hormonal Balance, Lower Blood Pressure, IBS, Cystitis, Varicose veins, Puffy eyes/Dark circles and Asthma.
  (NB: Roman Chamomile is better for mental & emotional problems (such as stress, anxiety etc). German Chamomile is better for physical problems (such as irritated skin).

3. FRANKINCENSE
is fabulous for the mind

> Chemical group: *Terpene*
> Price: *Inexpensive*
> Extraction: *Steam distillation of the resin of the tree/shrub*

BENEFITS:

- Can reduce symptoms of stress, anxiety, fear and grief.
- Can increase focus and creativity, and feelings of confidence and assertiveness.
- Can ease symptoms of Psoriasis/Eczema,
- Cystitis, Varicose Veins, Warts/Veruccas/Viral infections, Arthritis, Fertility/Hormonal Balance, Boosting the Immune & Respiratory Systems and reduces signs of ageing.

4. GERANIUM
is wonderful for hormonal problems, a true 'woman's oil'

> Chemical group: *Ester & Alcohol*
> Price: *Inexpensive*
> Extraction: *Steam distillation of the whole plant (leaves, flowers & stalks)*

BENEFITS:

- Can reduce symptoms of anxiety, depression, fear, rejection, anger, confusion, hurt and grief.
- Can increase positivity, relaxation and feelings of peace and contentment.
- Can uplift and ease symptoms of Menopause, PMT, Dry skin/Stretch marks, Fertility/Hormonal Balance, Varicose veins and Boosting the Immune System.

5. JASMINE
is perfect for emotional issues

> Chemical group: *Ester & Alcohol*
> Price: *Expensive*

Extraction: *Solvent extraction, Steam distillation, Enfleurage of the flowers*

BENEFITS:

- Can reduce depression, anxiety, regret, shame and guilt.

- Can increase positivity, confidence, assertiveness, relaxation and feelings of peace.

- Can ease symptoms of Menopause, PMT, Fertility/Hormonal Balance and reducing signs of ageing.

6. LAVENDER
is the best 'all-rounder' (panacea) oil

Chemical group: *Ester & Alcohol*
Price: *Inexpensive*
Extraction: *Steam distillation of the flowers*

BENEFITS:

- Can reduce symptoms of stress, anxiety, fear, depression and grief.

- Can increase relaxation and feelings of peace and contentment.

- Can ease symptoms of PMT, Menopause, Puffy eyes/Dark circles, Dry skin/Stretch marks, Psoriasis/Eczema, Aches/Pains (inc. headaches, arthritis), Relaxation, Lower Blood Pressure, Fertility/Hormonal Balance, Boosting Immune System, IBS, Cystitis, Varicose veins, Fungal infections, Coughs/Colds, Asthma and Snoring.

7. NEROLI
is a beautiful oil for the nervous system

Chemical group: *Alcohol & Terpene & Ester*
Price: *Expensive*

Extraction: *Solvent extraction, Steam distillation of orange blossom flowers*

BENEFITS:

- Can reduce symptoms of stress, anxiety, fear, grief and depression.

- Can increase positivity, relaxation and feelings of peace, joy and contentment.

- Can ease symptoms of PMT, Menopause, Psoriasis/Eczema, Varicose Veins, Boosting the Immune System and reducing signs of ageing.

8. ORANGE
is uplifting and soothing

Chemical group: *Terpene*
Price: *Inexpensive*
Extraction: *Expression of the rind/peel*

BENEFITS:

- Can reduce symptoms of anxiety, depression, fear, hurt and rejection.

- Can increase creativity, confidence, positivity and assertiveness.

- Can Aid relaxation, Lower blood pressure and Boost the Immune & Digestive Systems.

9. ROSE OTTO (AKA DAMASCENA (DAMASK)) OR ROSE ABSOLUTE (AKA CENTIFOLIA/MAROC/ROSE DE MAI (CABBAGE))
are wonderful for hormonal issues and emotional healing

Chemicals: *Alcohol & Terpene*

Price: *Expensive (Rose Otto is even more expensive than Rose Absolute)*
Extraction: *Steam distillation, Solvent extraction of the flower petals*

BENEFITS:

* Can reduce symptoms of grief, hurt, rejection, anxiety, fear and depression.

* Can increase confidence, positivity and assertiveness.

* Can ease symptoms of Psoriasis/Eczema, Fertility/Hormonal Balance, Puffy eyes/Dark circles, reducing signs of ageing.

10. YLANG YLANG
is a stress reducer and an aphrodisiac

Chemicals: *Ester & Alcohol & Terpene*
Price: *Inexpensive*
Extraction: *Steam distillation of the flower petals*

BENEFITS:

* Can reduce symptoms of depression, anxiety, fear, anger, guilt, regret and shame.

* Can increase confidence, assertiveness, focus and positivity.

* Can aid relaxation and ease symptoms of Psoriasis/Eczema, Fertility/Hormone Balance, Lower Blood Pressure and Boost the Immune System.

Only buy good quality essential oils, from reputable companies. You usually get what you pay for - so if the essential oils seem unusually cheap, they are probably not very good quality.

There are some essential oils which can cause problems for people with medical conditions (for example: diabetics, epileptics, heart disease/stroke patients).

The above listed essential oils are safe, but should only be used on healthy adults.

Except for Lavender and Tea Tree, no essential oils should be applied to the skin directly. Essential oils *must* be diluted in a Carrier Oil.

The 'Rescue Toolkit' carrier oils that every home should have:

1. GRAPE SEED
Inexpensive
Preferably for the body

BENEFITS:

* Fine texture, absorbs easily into the skin, almost odourless, suitable for all skin types including sensitive, tones and purifies the skin, contains Vitamin E, high fatty acid content which aids skin cell regeneration.

2. JOJOBA
Expensive
For the face or body

BENEFITS:

* Chemically similar to human sebum, is actually a wax not an oil and therefore is excellent for protecting and nourishing the skin, has a natural SPF5 good for all skin types including sensitive.

3. ROSEHIP
Expensive
Preferably for the face

BENEFITS:

• Excellent for treating skin conditions, stabilizing and strengthening for the skin, suitable for all skin types including sensitive, regenerates skin cells so is excellent for healing, one of the best oils for wrinkles.

4. EVENING PRIMROSE
Expensive
Preferably for the face

BENEFITS:

• Purifying, contains Omega 6 which is wonderful for relieving PMS/period pain, absorbs easily into the skin, very nourishing.

5. SUNFLOWER
Inexpensive
For face or body

BENEFITS:

• Absorbs quickly into the skin, contains more Vitamin E than any other carrier oil, softens the skin, good for all skin types including sensitive.

How to make a Safely Diluted Massage Blend:

"**2% Blend**" = 2 drops of essential oil into/per 5ml of carrier oil (up to a maximum of 8 drops into 20ml carrier oil) . This blend is for HEALTHY ADULTS, and is for use on the BODY.
"**1% Blend**" = 1 drop of essential oil into/per 5ml of carrier oil (up to a maximum of 4 drops into 20ml carrier oil). This blend is for CHILDREN (over 11 years) & ELDERLY, and is for use on the BODY.

When creating a Blend for the FACE, only use a "**1% Blend**"

Use up to **three essential oils** MAXIMUM per blend (and split the maximum drops of essential oil BETWEEN these three)

Important Safety Disclaimer:
For the purposes of this book, do NOT use essential oils on babies/children, adults who are ill (including seriously ill), the elderly, and pregnant/breastfeeding women.
(*Essential oils can be used on the aforementioned people, but only by professionally **qualified aromatherapists**).*

How to Personalise your Blend:
Incorporate up to 3 oils in a blend that cover your:
1. Physical need
2. Mental need
3. Emotional need at that moment.

You may find that only one particular oil is perfect for all three needs, and that is fine.
Use essential oils that you like the smell of, not just because of their therapeutic benefits. If you do not like the smell(s), your body will counteract any therapeutic benefit you would have gained.

OTHER WAYS OF USING ESSENTIAL OILS:

BATH
Pour a teaspoon of your Blend into a warm bath.
<u>Caution:</u> Take extra care when entering/exiting the
bath, as the Blend may make it **slippery**.
Alternatively, disperse 6 drops of essential oil in half
a cup of full fat milk (approx 120ml) and add to a
warm bath.

SHOWER
Put a few drops of pure essential oil (**<u>not</u>** your Blend,
as this will be <u>slippery</u>) on the floor of the shower,
cover the drain and inhale the aroma whilst
showering.

HANDKERCHIEF/FLANNEL
Put a few drops of pure essential oil (not a Blend)
onto a tissue/handkerchief/flannel and inhale.

HOT COMPRESS
Fill a bowl with 500ml hot water
Add 6 drops of essential oil
Carefully place a folded piece of sterile cotton cloth
into the fragranced water
Carefully squeeze out any excess water
Place the moistened cloth onto the affected body
area until it reaches body temperature
Repeat steps 3 through 5 two to three times
*Hot compresses are helpful for backaches,
rheumatism, arthritis, period pain.*

COLD COMPRESS
Fill a bowl with 500ml ice cold water
Add 6 drops of essential oil
Carefully place a folded piece of sterile cotton cloth
into the fragranced water
Carefully squeeze out any excess water
Place the moistened cloth onto the affected body
area until it reaches body temperature
Repeat steps 3 through 5 two to three times
*Cold compresses are helpful for headaches, neck
tension, varicose veins, sprains and strains.*

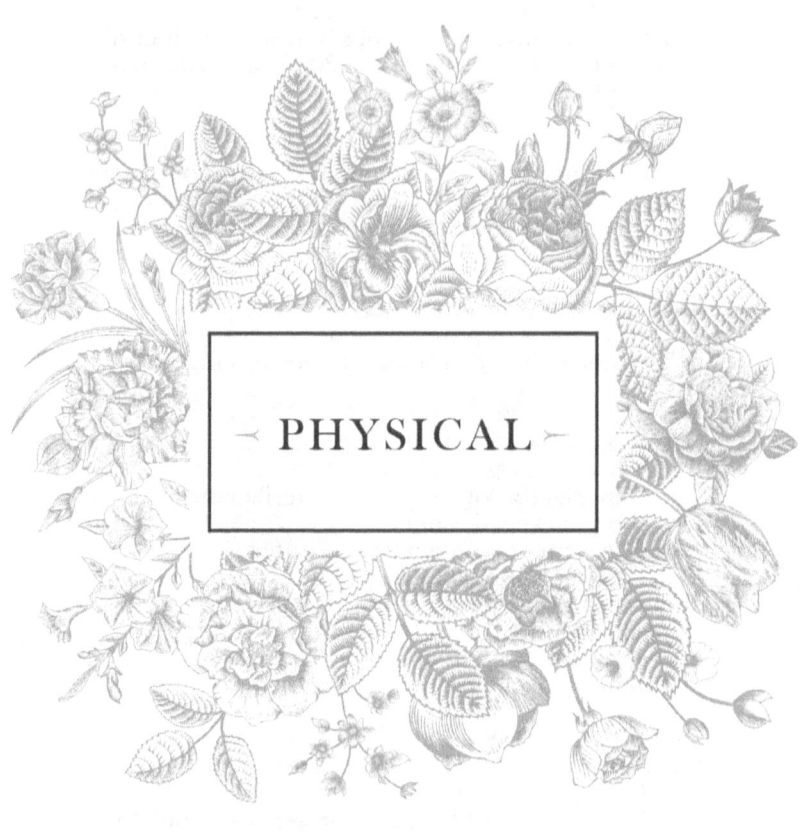

PHYSICAL

4

BEST ESSENTIAL OILS
FOR ANTI-AGEING

From your 'Rescue Toolkit' essential oils:

Bergamot	Lavender
Chamomile	Neroli
Frankincense	Rose
Geranium	Ylang Ylang
Jasmine	

ADDITIONAL ESSENTIAL OILS:

Palmarosa	Rosewood
Patchouli	Sandalwood

Firming the skin: Frankincense, Lavender, Neroli
Usage: 1% Facial Massage Blend. See notes on 'Your
Rescue Kit & How to Create a Blend'.

**Reducing Wrinkles & fine lines/Plumping
the skin:** Geranium, Neroli, Palmarosa, Patchouli,
Rose, Sandalwood
Usage: 1% Facial Massage Blend. See notes on 'Your

Rescue Kit & How to Create a Blend'.

Age spots/Lightening the skin: Bergamot, Chamomile, Frankincense, Geranium, Lavender, Ylang Ylang
Usage: 1% Facial Massage Blend. See notes on 'Your Rescue Kit & How to Create a Blend'.

Broken Capillaries/Thread veins: Frankincense, Geranium, Lavender, Rose, Ylang Ylang
Usage: 1% Facial Massage Blend. See notes on 'Your Rescue Kit & How to Create a Blend'.

Lifting/Toning the skin: Geranium, Frankincense, Lavender, Rose, Rosewood
Usage: 1% Facial Massage Blend. See notes on 'Your Rescue Kit & How to Create a Blend'.

Reducing Dullness/Brightening the skin/For Radiance: Frankincense, Geranium, Lavender, Sandalwood
Usage: 1% Facial Massage Blend. See notes on 'Your Rescue Kit & How to Create a Blend'.

Puffy eyes/Dark circles: Chamomile, Lavender, Patchouli, Rose.
Usage: 1% Facial Massage Blend. See notes on 'Your Rescue Kit & How to Create a Blend'.

Also try using cooled Chamomile teabags or cucumber slices or Rosewater soaked cotton pads placed onto eyelids.

Reduce caffeine & alcohol intake.

If having more sleep doesn't seem to help reduce the puffiness/dark circles, try cutting out wheat for one week too.

FROM YOUR 'RECOMMENDED CARRIER OILS':

GRAPE SEED
Inexpensive

BENEFITS:
Fine texture, absorbs easily into the skin, almost odourless, suitable for all skin types including sensitive, tones and purifies the skin, high fatty acid content which aids skin cell regeneration.

JOJOBA
Expensive

BENEFITS:
Chemically similar to human sebum, is actually a wax not an oil and therefore is excellent for protecting and nourishing the skin, has a natural SPF5 good for all skin types including sensitive.

ROSEHIP
Expensive

BENEFITS:
Excellent for treating skin conditions, stabilizing and strengthening for the skin, suitable for all skin types including sensitive, regenerates skin cells so is excellent for healing, one of the best oils for wrinkles.

ADDITIONAL 'FATTY' CARRIER OILS:

ARGAN
Expensive

BENEFITS:
Contains Vitamin E and antioxidants which are excellent for anti-ageing, healing for skin conditions.

COCONUT

Inexpensive

BENEFITS:
Odourless, non irritant, nourishing.

OLIVE
Inexpensive

BENEFITS:
High vitamin and mineral content, quality lubricant, but has an odour.

ADDITIONAL ADVICE:

- Use a body exfoliator/scrub to get rid of dead skin cells (maximum twice a week), before applying your Blend to your body - this will ensure that the 'goodness' from your blend penetrates the skin more readily.

- Use a facial exfoliator/scrub to get rid of dead skin cells (maximum twice a week), before applying your Blend to your face - this will ensure that the 'goodness' from your blend penetrates the skin more readily. Do **not** exfoliate Rosecea or very Sensitive skin though.
  Use a **1% BLEND** ON THE FACE (*See notes on 'Your Rescue Kit & How to Create a Blend'*).

- Increase your intake of dark berries (e.g.: Blackberries), dark chocolate, green leafy vegetables (e.g.: spinach), tomatoes and citrus fruits, which are all high in **antioxidants**.

- Increase your intake of **Vitamins & Minerals** - by eating more brown rice and oats.

- Increase your intake of **Omega 3** - by eating more salmon, sardines, tuna and kidney beans.

- Increase your intake of **Vitamin E** - by eating more avocados and/or taking Vitamin E supplements (using the manufacturer's instructions).

• Vitamin E is a fabulous ingredient for improving and protecting the skin. Many skin care companies use it in their products, so seek out/use those that do.

• Ensure that your skin care products contain Vitamin A, as this is one of the most important anti-ageing ingredients.

• Wear a sunscreen lotion/cream whenever possible.

5

BEST ESSENTIAL OILS
FOR
PAIN MANAGEMENT

From your 'Rescue Toolkit' essential oils:

Bergamot   Lavender
Chamomile   Neroli
Frankincense

ADDITIONAL ESSENTIAL OILS:

Marjoram   Tea Tree
Peppermint

HEADACHES/MIGRAINES
Chamomile, Lavender, Peppermint

Usage: 1% Massage Blend, Cold Compress. See notes on 'Your Rescue Kit & How to Create a Blend'.

INFLAMMATORY PAIN (INC. ARTHRITIS/JOINT PAIN/GOUT)
Chamomile, Frankincense, Lavender, Marjoram, Peppermint, Tea Tree

Usage: Bath, Hot Compress. See notes on 'Your Rescue Kit & How to Create a Blend'.

MUSCLE ACHES/PAINS
Chamomile, Lavender, Marjoram

Usage: Bath, Hot Compress. See notes on 'Your Rescue Kit & How to Create a Blend'.

MENSTRUAL CRAMPS/PERIOD PAIN/PMT
Bergamot, Chamomile, Geranium, Lavender, Marjoram, Neroli

Usage: Bath, Hot Compress. See notes on 'Your Rescue Kit & How to Create a Blend'.

FROM YOUR 'RECOMMENDED CARRIER OILS':

EVENING PRIMROSE
Expensive
Preferably for the face

BENEFITS:
Purifying, contains Omega 6 which is wonderful for relieving PMS/period pain, absorbs easily into the skin, very nourishing.

ROSEHIP
Expensive
Preferably for the face

BENEFITS:
Excellent for treating skin conditions, stabilizing and strengthening for the skin, suitable for all skin types including sensitive, regenerates skin cells so is excellent

for healing, one of the best oils for wrinkles.

SUNFLOWER
Inexpensive
For face or body

BENEFITS:
Absorbs quickly into the skin, contains more Vitamin E than any other carrier oil, softens the skin, good for all skin types including sensitive.

Instead of creating/using an oil 'Blend', there may be times when a compress is more effective for pain relief. See notes for 'Your Rescue Kit & How to Create a Blend'.

ADDITIONAL ADVICE:

FOR SUFFERERS OF HEADACHES/MIGRAINES:

• Try eating a gluten free diet (inc. avoiding eating wheat, rye & oats) for two weeks to see if there is any difference (as gluten can trigger headaches).

• Avoid chocolate, cheese, red wine, coffee and tea (as they contain natural substances called vasoactive amines, which can trigger headaches).

• Eat more almonds and avocados (which contain high levels of Vitamin E). Vitamin E is a vasodilator and widens the blood vessels, which in turn thins blood and allows it to flow more freely around the body, therefore unblocking tension.

FOR SUFFERERS OF PERIOD PAIN:

- Avoid refined carbohydrates, instead eat more whole grains like oats, brown rice and quinoa.

- Eliminate sugary foods and processed sugar.

- Reduce/eliminate dairy products as they are congesting to the body. If you do choose dairy, at least try to purchase organic, in order to avoid added hormones.

- Reduce your intake of red meat and egg yolk. Or at least choose organic free range meats and eggs when possible, to avoid added hormones.

- Eat more fresh fruits and vegetables.

6

BEST ESSENTIAL OILS
FOR RELAXATION
& ENERGIZING

From your 'Rescue Toolkit' essential oils:

Bergamot   Neroli
Chamomile   Orange
Frankincense   Rose
Geranium   Ylang Ylang
Lavender

ADDITIONAL ESSENTIAL OILS:

Marjoram
Peppermint

ESSENTIAL OILS FOR THE
RELAXATION CATEGORY:
*(**Avoid** these oils if you have LOW Blood Pressure)*

ADHD
Frankincense, Lavender, Vetiver

HIGH BLOOD PRESSURE (HYPERTENSION)
Lavender, Marjoram, Ylang Ylang

TO RELAX THE BODY IN GENERAL
Bergamot, Chamomile, Geranium, Lavender,
Marjoram, Neroli, Orange, Rose, Ylang Ylang

Usage:
Either massage your Blend into your skin, or
alternatively, use a small amount in the bath (**taking
extra care** as you get in/out of the bath, as it may
be slippery).
See notes on 'Your Rescue Kit & How to Create a
Blend'.

ESSENTIAL OILS FOR THE
ENERGISING CATEGORY:
*(**Avoid** these oils if you have HIGH Blood Pressure)*

OVERCOMING PHYSICAL TIREDNESS
Bergamot, Orange, Geranium, Peppermint

LOW BLOOD PRESSURE (HYPOTENSION)
Geranium, Peppermint

Usage:
Massage your Blend into your skin, or alternatively,
use 3 drops of essential oils onto a flannel in the

shower, to 'wake you up'.

You can also put a few drops of pure essential oil (**not** your Blend, as this will be <u>slippery</u>) onto the floor of your shower, cover the drain and inhale the aroma whilst showering.

See notes on 'Your Rescue Kit & How to Create a Blend'.

From your 'Recommended Carrier Oils':

Grape seed
Inexpensive
Preferably for the body

BENEFITS:
Fine texture, absorbs easily into the skin, almost odourless, suitable for all skin types including sensitive, tones and purifies the skin, high fatty acid content which aids skin cell regeneration.

Jojoba
Expensive
For the face or body

BENEFITS:
Chemically similar to human sebum, is actually a wax not an oil and therefore is excellent for protecting and nourishing the skin, has a natural SPF5 good for all skin types including sensitive.

Sunflower
Inexpensive

For face or body

BENEFITS:
Absorbs quickly into the skin, contains more Vitamin
E than any other carrier oil, softens the skin, good
for all skin types including sensitive.

ADDITIONAL ADVICE:

FOODS WHICH HELP YOU TO RELAX:

Asparagus - Vitamin B
Avocados - Potassium, Glutathione, Folate
Bananas - Potassium
Carrots/Celery (crunchy veg) - Nutrients
Low fat milk - Protein, B Vitamins, Vitamin D
Chamomile Tea
Egg yolks - Choline
Salmon/Sardines/Tuna (fatty fish) - Omega 3 fatty
acids
Dark chocolate (70% cacao content or more + with
as little added sugar as possible) - reduces stress
hormones

FOODS WHICH HELP TO GIVE YOU ENERGY:

Pumpkin/Sunflower seeds - Magnesium
Green tea - Caffeine, Antioxidants
Citrus fruits, strawberries, mangoes, apricots, kiwi -
Vitamin C
Spinach/Kale - Vitamins, Iron, Magnesium
Lean meat - Protein, Vitamin B12
Eggs - Minerals, Protein
Yoghurt - B Vitamins

7

BEST ESSENTIAL OILS
FOR SKIN PROBLEMS

From your 'Rescue Toolkit' essential oils:

Bergamot   Lavender
Chamomile   Neroli
Frankincense   Orange
Geranium   Rose
Jasmine   Ylang Ylang

ADDITIONAL ESSENTIAL OILS:

Benzoin   Patchouli
Carrot Seed   Palmarosa
Mandarin   Rosewood

SENSITIVE SKIN
Chamomile, Jasmine, Lavender, Neroli, Palmarosa,
Rose, Rosewood

Usage: 1% Facial Massage Blend. See notes on 'Your Rescue Kit & How to Create a Blend'.

DRY SKIN
Benzoin, Carrot Seed, Chamomile, Geranium, Jasmine, Lavender, Mandarin, Neroli, Patchouli, Rose

Usage: 1% Facial Massage Blend. See notes on 'Your Rescue Kit & How to Create a Blend'.

OILY SKIN
Bergamot, Chamomile, Frankincense, Geranium, Lavender, Patchouli, Rose, Rosewood, Ylang Ylang

Usage: 1% Facial Massage Blend. See notes on 'Your Rescue Kit & How to Create a Blend'.

ACNE SKIN
Bergamot, Chamomile, Geranium, Lavender, Palmarosa, Rosewood, Ylang Ylang

Usage: 1% Facial Massage Blend. See notes on 'Your Rescue Kit & How to Create a Blend'.

HORMONAL SKIN
Chamomile, Frankincense, Geranium, Rose

Usage: 1% Facial Massage Blend. See notes on 'Your Rescue Kit & How to Create a Blend'.

ROSACEA
Chamomile, Frankincense, Lavender

Usage: 1% Facial Massage Blend. See notes on 'Your Rescue Kit & How to Create a Blend'.

CELLULITE
Geranium, Mandarin, Orange

Usage: 2% (Body) Massage Blend. See notes on 'Your Rescue Kit & How to Create a Blend'.

STRETCH MARKS
Benzoin, Geranium, Lavender, Mandarin, Patchouli

Usage: 2% (Body) Massage Blend. See notes on 'Your Rescue Kit & How to Create a Blend'.

AGE SPOTS
Bergamot, Chamomile, Frankincense, Geranium, Lavender, Ylang Ylang

Usage: 1% Facial Massage Blend. See notes on 'Your Rescue Kit & How to Create a Blend'.

BROKEN CAPILLARIES
Frankincense, Geranium, Lavender, Ylang Ylang

Usage: 1% Facial Massage Blend. See notes on 'Your Rescue Kit & How to Create a Blend'.

PSORIASIS
Bergamot, Benzoin, Chamomile, Frankincense, Lavender, Neroli, Rose, Rosewood, Ylang Ylang

Usage: 2% (Body) Massage Blend. See notes on 'Your Rescue Kit & How to Create a Blend'.

ECZEMA
Benzoin, Chamomile, Frankincense, Lavender, Neroli, Palmarosa, Rose, Rosewood, Ylang Ylang

Usage: 2% (Body) Massage Blend. See notes on 'Your Rescue Kit & How to Create a Blend'.

From your 'Recommended Carrier Oils':

Grape seed
Inexpensive
Preferably for the body

BENEFITS:
Fine texture, absorbs easily into the skin, almost odourless, suitable for all skin types including sensitive, tones and purifies the skin, high fatty acid content which aids skin cell regeneration.

Rosehip
Expensive
Preferably for the face

BENEFITS:
Excellent for treating skin conditions, stabilizing and strengthening for the skin, suitable for all skin types including sensitive, regenerates skin cells so is excellent for healing, one of the best oils for wrinkles.

Jojoba
Expensive
For the face or body

BENEFITS:
Chemically similar to human sebum, is actually a wax not an oil and therefore is excellent for protecting and nourishing the skin, has a natural SPF5 good for all skin types including sensitive.

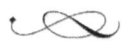

ADDITIONAL 'FATTY' CARRIER OILS:

COCONUT
Inexpensive
Preferably for the body

BENEFITS:
Odourless, non irritant, nourishing.

OLIVE
Inexpensive

BENEFITS:
High vitamin and mineral content, quality lubricant, but has an odour.

ADDITIONAL ADVICE:

*   Use a body exfoliator/scrub to get rid of dead skin cells (maximum twice a week), before applying your Blend to your body - this will ensure that the 'goodness' from your blend penetrates the skin more readily.

*   Use a facial exfoliator/scrub to get rid of dead skin cells (maximum twice a week), before applying your Blend to your face - this will ensure that the 'goodness' from your blend penetrates the skin more readily.

*   Do **not** exfoliate Rosecea or very Sensitive skin though. USE A **1% BLEND** ON THE FACE (*See notes on 'Your Rescue Kit & How to Create a Blend'*).

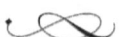

IF YOU ARE TRYING TO REMOVE/SOFTEN HARD, DRY SKIN FROM YOUR FEET, THIS ROUTINE WILL HELP:

- Soak your feet in warm water
- Use a body exfoliator/scrub or a pumice to remove dead/hard skin
- Smooth on your Blend (or a thick layer of nourishing foot cream etc) all over your feet
- Individually wrap your feet in cling film/saran wrap (yes, you heard me correctly!)
- Now put on a thick, warm pair of socks
- Leave them on for at least half an hour (some people leave overnight)
- When you've removed the socks and cling film, massage in any remaining Blend or cream
- Repeat this process twice a week
- The heat generated from the cling film & socks, plus the fact that you've exfoliated, ensures that the oil/cream deeply penetrate your skin, and will leave them soft and nourished!
- Increase your intake of Vitamin E - by eating more avocados and/or taking **Vitamin E** supplements (using the manufacturer's instructions).
- Increase your intake of **Zinc** - by eating more chicken, natural yoghurt and brown rice.
- Increase your intake of **Omega 3** - by eating more salmon, sardines, tuna and kidney beans.
- Vitamin E is a fabulous ingredient for improving and protecting the skin. Seek out skin care products which include Vitamin E in their ingredients list.

8

BEST ESSENTIAL OILS
FOR SPECIFIC
HEALTH AILMENTS

From your 'Rescue Toolkit' essential oils:

Bergamot   Lavender
Chamomile   Neroli
Frankincense   Orange
Geranium   Ylang Ylang

ADDITIONAL ESSENTIAL OILS:

Grapefruit   Peppermint
Mandarin   Rosewood
Marjoram   Sandalwood
Palmarosa   Tea Tree
Patchouli

BOOST IMMUNE SYSTEM (INC. LUPUS, THYROID PROBLEMS, DIABETES, MULTIPLE SCLEROSIS)
Bergamot, Chamomile, Frankincense, Geranium, Lavender, Marjoram, Neroli, Orange, Sandalwood, Ylang Ylang

Usage: Massage Blend. See notes on 'Your Rescue Kit & How to Create a Blend'.

IBS
Chamomile, Frankincense, Lavender, Marjoram, Peppermint

Usage: Massage Blend, or pour small amount of the Massage Blend into a warm bath, or disperse essential oils into milk and pour into bath. See notes on 'Your Rescue Kit & How to Create a Blend'.

Also: try drinking Peppermint Tea.

CYSTITIS
Bergamot, Chamomile, Frankincense, Lavender, Rosewood, Sandalwood, Tea Tree

Usage: Hot compress or Massage Blend. See notes on 'Your Rescue Kit & How to Create a Blend'.

VARICOSE VEINS
Bergamot, Chamomile, Frankincense, Geranium, Lavender, Neroli, Palmarosa

Usage: Cold Compress. See notes on 'Your Rescue Kit & How to Create a Blend'.

FUNGAL INFECTIONS (ATHLETES FOOT, RINGWORM, YEAST INFECTIONS)
Lavender, Tea Tree

Usage: Massage Blend. See notes on 'Your Rescue Kit & How to Create a Blend'.

VIRAL INFECTIONS (INC. WARTS, VERUCCAS)
Bergamot, Frankincense, Tea Tree

Usage: Massage Blend. See notes on 'Your Rescue Kit & How to Create a Blend'.

COUGHS/COLDS
Lavender, Tea Tree

Usage: Put a few drops of pure essential oil (not a Blend) onto a tissue/handkerchief and inhale, or put a few drops of pure essential oil (**not** your Blend, as this will be slippery) on the floor of the shower, cover the drain and inhale the aroma whilst showering.

SNORING
Lavender, Marjoram, Peppermint

Usage: Put a few drops of pure essential oil (not a Blend) onto a tissue/handkerchief, place on pillow and inhale.

WEIGHT LOSS (INC. INCREASING METABOLISM/TONING/REDUCING CELLULITE & STRETCH MARKS/REDUCING APPETITE & STRESS TRIGGERED EATING, PREVENTING WATER RETENTION & BLOATING. AIDING DIGESTION)
Bergamot, Geranium, Grapefruit, Lavender, Peppermint, Sandalwood

Usage: Massage Blend. See notes on 'Your Rescue Kit

& How to Create a Blend'.

DETOX (INC. HANGOVER)
Peppermint, Grapefruit, Lavender, Mandarin,
Orange, Patchouli

Usage: Massage Blend or Cold Compress. See notes
on 'Your Rescue Kit & How to Create a Blend'.

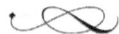

FROM YOUR 'RECOMMENDED CARRIER OILS':

GRAPE SEED
Inexpensive
Preferably for the body

BENEFITS:
Fine texture, absorbs easily into the skin, almost
odourless, suitable for all skin types including
sensitive, tones and purifies the skin, high fatty acid
content which aids skin cell regeneration.

JOJOBA
Expensive
For the face or body

BENEFITS:
Chemically similar to human sebum, is actually a wax
not an oil and therefore is excellent for protecting
and nourishing the skin, has a natural SPF5 good for
all skin types including sensitive.

SUNFLOWER
Inexpensive
For face or body

BENEFITS:
Absorbs quickly into the skin, contains more Vitamin
E than any other carrier oil, softens the skin, good
for all skin types including sensitive.

9

BEST ESSENTIAL OILS
FOR WOMEN'S ISSUES

From your 'Rescue Toolkit' essential oils:

Bergamot	Lavender
Chamomile	Neroli
Frankincense	Rose
Geranium	Ylang Ylang

ADDITIONAL ESSENTIAL OILS:

Jasmine	Marjoram

MENSTRUAL CRAMPS/PERIOD PAIN/PMT:
*Bergamot, Chamomile, Geranium, Lavender,
Marjoram, Neroli*

Usage: Bath, Hot Compress or Massage Blend. See
notes on 'Your Rescue Kit & How to Create a Blend'.

MENOPAUSE:

Chamomile, Geranium, Jasmine, Lavender, Neroli

Usage: Bath, Massage Blend or Cold Compress (for sweating/hot flushes). See notes on 'Your Rescue Kit & How to Create a Blend'.

FERTILITY/HORMONAL BALANCE:
Chamomile, Frankincense, Geranium, Jasmine, Lavender, Marjoram, Rose Otto, Ylang Ylang

Usage: Massage Blend (get your partner to massage you for added romance!). See notes on 'Your Rescue Kit & How to Create a Blend'.

FROM YOUR 'RECOMMENDED CARRIER OILS':

GRAPE SEED
Inexpensive
Preferably for the body

BENEFITS:
Fine texture, absorbs easily into the skin, almost odourless, suitable for all skin types including sensitive, tones and purifies the skin, high fatty acid content which aids skin cell regeneration.

EVENING PRIMROSE
Expensive
Preferably for the face

BENEFITS:
Purifying, contains Omega 6 which is wonderful for relieving PMS/period pain, absorbs easily into the skin, very nourishing.

SUNFLOWER
Inexpensive
For face or body

BENEFITS:
Absorbs quickly into the skin, contains more Vitamin E than any other carrier oil, softens the skin, good for all skin types including sensitive.

ADDITIONAL INFORMATION:

FOR PMT/MENSTRUAL CRAMPS/PERIOD PAIN:

- Avoid refined carbohydrates, instead eat more whole grains like oats, brown rice and quinoa.

- Eliminate sugary foods and processed sugar.

- Reduce/eliminate dairy products as they are congesting to the body.
  If you do choose dairy, at least try to purchase organic, in order to avoid added hormones.

- Reduce your intake of red meat and egg yolk. Or at least choose organic free range meats and eggs when possible, to avoid added hormones.

- Eat more fresh fruits and vegetables.

FOR MENOPAUSE:

- Increase calcium intake (dairy products, yoghurt, salmon, sardines) which help with bone health.

- Increase iron intake (poultry, fish, eggs, leafy green vegetables).

- Increase fibre intake (whole-grain breads, cereals, pasta, rice, fresh fruits and vegetables).

- Increase the amount of water you drink.

- Eat pumpkin/sunflower/sesame seeds, which have high levels of Vitamin E, zinc and calcium. These normalize hormone levels and prevent dry skin.

- Eat more turkey, cottage cheese and oats, which manufacture serotonin (to help with depression/mood swings).

- Reduce fat intake, which can lead to weight gain (e.g.: fatty meats, whole milk, ice cream and cheese).

- Reduce salt and sugar intake (which can add to feelings of tiredness and lead to weight gain).

- Reduce stimulants such as alcohol, spicy food, chocolate (which can increase hot flushes).

FOR FERTILITY:

Avoid:
- Red meat

- Refined sugar

- Non-organic chicken

- Refined carbohydrates (white bread, sugar and rice)

Reduce:
- Alcohol and caffeine.

Increase intake of:
- Bananas (Vitamin B6)

- Asparagus (Folic Acid)

- Eggs (Vitamin D, Protein)

- Citrus Fruits (Vitamin C)

- Chicken/Turkey (Iron, Protein)

- Peas (Zinc)
- Salmon/Cod/Mackerel (Omega 3 Fatty Acids, Protein)
- Fruits & Vegetables (Antioxidants, Fibre)
- Sunflower Seeds (Zinc)
- Pumpkin Seeds (Iron)
- Broccoli/Spinach/Dark Green Leafy Vegetables (phytosterols, fibre, magnesium)
- Complex Carbohydrates (e.g.: brown rice, wholegrains)

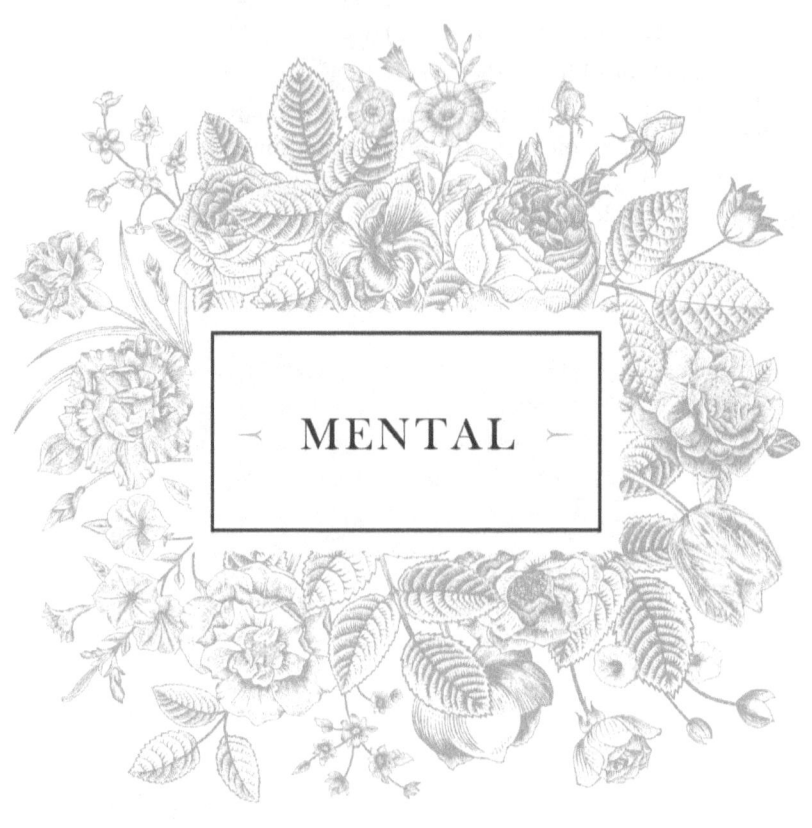

MENTAL

10

BEST ESSENTIAL OILS
FOR DEPRESSION

From your 'Rescue Toolkit' essential oils:

Bergamot	Lavender
Chamomile	Neroli
Frankincense	Orange
Geranium	Rose
Jasmine	Ylang Ylang

ADDITIONAL ESSENTIAL OILS:

Marjoram	Sandalwood
Petitgrain	

Usage: Massage, Bath, Shower, Handkerchief/Flannel. See notes on 'Your Rescue Kit & How to Create a Blend'.

FROM YOUR 'RECOMMENDED CARRIER OILS':

GRAPE SEED
Inexpensive

Preferably for the body

BENEFITS:
Fine texture, absorbs easily into the skin, almost odourless, suitable for all skin types including sensitive, tones and purifies the skin, high fatty acid content which aids skin cell regeneration.

JOJOBA
Expensive
For the face or body

BENEFITS:
Chemically similar to human sebum, is actually a wax not an oil and therefore is excellent for protecting and nourishing the skin, has a natural SPF5 good for all skin types including sensitive.

SUNFLOWER
Inexpensive
For face or body

BENEFITS:
Absorbs quickly into the skin, contains more Vitamin E than any other carrier oil, softens the skin, good for all skin types including sensitive.

ADDITIONAL ADVICE:

As well as any relevant medication and/or counselling you may be receiving:

• Eat more vitamin and antioxidant rich foods, such as apricots, broccoli, carrots, spinach, sweet potatoes, blueberries, oranges, peppers, tomatoes, sunflower seeds, vegetable oils.

• Eat complex carbohydrates, such as whole grains.

- Eat protein rich foods, such as poultry, tuna, beans/peas, lean beef, fish, low fat dairy products.

- Reduce your intake of caffeine, sugar and alcohol.

- Drink more water.

- Exercise, in particular exercising outside of your home (gym, walk in the park etc).

- Try to get out in the sunshine as much as possible/time in nature.

- Cultivate supportive relationships (family, friends, support groups etc - especially with positive people).

- Get enough sleep (approx 8 hours).

- Practice relaxation techniques (meditation is a great example).

- Do things you enjoy (examples may include: art, listening to/play music, dance, listening to motivational/inspirational/spiritual cd's, theatre trips, travel, coffee with friends, hobbies, sport, reading, watching a funny film, playing with a pet).

This information is intended to complement medical treatment/medication, not as a replacement.

11

BEST ESSENTIAL OILS
FOR INSOMNIA

From your 'Rescue Toolkit' essential oils:

Chamomile   Neroli
Lavender

ADDITIONAL ESSENTIAL OILS:

Marjoram   Sandalwood
Patchouli   Vetiver

Usage: Massage, Bath, Handkerchief (to then place on pillow).

See notes on 'Your Rescue Kit & How to Create a Blend'.

FROM YOUR 'RECOMMENDED CARRIER OILS':

GRAPE SEED
Inexpensive

Preferably for the body

BENEFITS:
Fine texture, absorbs easily into the skin, almost
odourless, suitable for all skin types including
sensitive, tones and purifies the skin, high fatty acid
content which aids skin cell regeneration.

JOJOBA
Expensive
For the face or body

BENEFITS:
Chemically similar to human sebum, is actually a wax
not an oil and therefore is excellent for protecting
and nourishing the skin, has a natural SPF5 good for
all skin types including sensitive.

SUNFLOWER
Inexpensive
For face or body

BENEFITS:
Absorbs quickly into the skin, contains more Vitamin
E than any other carrier oil, softens the skin, good
for all skin types including sensitive.

ADDITIONAL ADVICE:

Increasing your serotonin levels can help to aid
sleep, some ways of doing this are:

- Eat more complex carbohydrates (such as
  oatmeal, quinoa, barley, sweet potatoes and
  whole grain bread), including for dinner.

- Eat more turkey.

- Eat more bananas.

- Also, try drinking Chamomile tea/Valerian tea/warm milk before bed, as opposed to caffeine and/or alcohol.

- Increase your iron intake by eating lean red meat (for lunch, not dinner).

12

BEST ESSENTIAL OILS
FOR MENTAL FATIGUE
& CONCENTRATION

From your 'Rescue Toolkit' essential oils:

Bergamot   Lavender
Frankincense   Neroli
Geranium   Orange
Jasmine

ADDITIONAL ESSENTIAL OILS:

Peppermint

MENTAL FATIGUE & TIREDNESS/ BURN OUT
Bergamot, Frankincense, Jasmine, Lavender, Neroli, Orange, Peppermint

Usage: Massage or Inhalation (via shower or flannel/handkerchief). See notes for 'Your Rescue Kit & How to Create a Blend').

ME (CHRONIC FATIGUE SYNDROME)
Frankincense, Geranium, Lavender, Orange

Usage: Massage or Inhalation (via shower or flannel/handkerchief). See notes for 'Your Rescue Kit & How to Create a Blend').

CONCENTRATION
Frankincense, Orange, Peppermint

Usage: Massage or Inhalation (via shower or flannel/handkerchief). See notes for 'Your Rescue Kit & How to Create a Blend').

FROM YOUR 'RECOMMENDED CARRIER OILS':

EVENING PRIMROSE
Expensive
Preferably for the face

BENEFITS:
Purifying, contains Omega 6 which is wonderful for relieving PMS/period pain, absorbs easily into the skin, very nourishing.

ROSEHIP
Expensive
Preferably for the face

BENEFITS:
Excellent for treating skin conditions, stabilizing and strengthening for the skin, suitable for all skin types including sensitive, regenerates skin cells so is excellent for healing, one of the best oils for wrinkles.

SUNFLOWER
Inexpensive
For face or body

BENEFITS:
Absorbs quickly into the skin, contains more Vitamin E than any other carrier oil, softens the skin, good for all skin types including sensitive.
Additional advice:

FOR MENTAL FATIGUE & TIREDNESS/ BURN OUT:

- Eat more complex carbohydrates such as whole grain breads, sweet potatoes and brown rice.

- Eat more unsaturated fats and protein (e.g.: tuna, carrots).

- Eat more iron-rich food source, such as lentils, soybeans or lean red meat.

- To help absorb iron better, eat more vitamin C sources, such as oranges, broccoli/vegetables.

- Eat more protein, such as yogurt, cottage cheese, low-fat cheese, chicken, fish, turkey.

- Drink green tea and more water.

FOR ME (CHRONIC FATIGUE SYNDROME):

- Eat animal-based proteins, such as milk, meat, fish, poultry and eggs.

- Eat complex carbohydrates, such as grains and beans.

- Eat (small amounts of) dark chocolate (which gives a moderate amount of caffeine).

- Eat more protein, such as poultry, fish, lean meats or dried beans.

- Eat dairy products, such as low-fat milk, cheese or yogurt.

- Eat more fruit and vegetables, such as avocados.

- Eat foods which contain Omega 3's, such as mackerel, salmon, trout and sardines.

- Avoid high calorie foods, fried foods/high saturated fats, refined sugar, MSG, cigarettes/tobacco, caffeine, alcohol.

FOR CONCENTRATION:

- Eat foods which contain Omega 3's, such as mackerel, salmon, trout and sardines.

- Eat foods high in antioxidants (vitamins A, C, E) such as berries (especially blueberries), tomatoes, cauliflower, cabbage and broccoli.

- Try green tea and dark chocolate which give moderate amounts of caffeine and antioxidants.

- Also try drinking peppermint tea, and more water.

- Eat foods which are high in B6 & B12 such as fish, meat, whole grains, eggs and dairy (such as low fat yoghurt).

- Eat foods high in fibre such as vegetables, fruits (such as bananas), whole grains, seeds (such as sunflower, and is also high in Vitamin E) and beans.

13

BEST ESSENTIAL OILS
FOR STRESS,
ANXIETY & FEAR

This one of the **most important** chapters to remember, because essential oils for these conditions are the *most commonly requested*. In fact, almost every other (physical, mental, emotional) condition mentioned in this book is linked to either stress, anxiety or fear (or any combination of them).

The fact is, stress is not a REAL thing - it is only our perception/judgment of a situation. This 'stress' can only be relieved by changing our thoughts. However, our negative ('stressful') thoughts do have the *potential* to then manifest as bodily ailments, and the oils below can help to ease this pain and help your mind & body to relax.

From your 'Rescue Toolkit' essential oils:

Bergamot   Geranium
Chamomile   Jasmine
Frankincense   Lavender

Neroli   Ylang Ylang
Rose Otto

ADDITIONAL ESSENTIAL OILS:

Benzoin   Sandalwood
Melissa   Vetiver
Rosewood

EXCESS, NEGATIVE STRESS:

Bergamot, Chamomile, Frankincense, Geranium, Jasmine, Lavender, Marjoram, Melissa, Neroli, Orange, Patchouli, Rose, Sandalwood, Vetiver, Ylang Ylang

Usage: Massage, Bath or Handkerchief/Flannel. See notes on 'Your Rescue Kit & How to Create a Blend'.

ANXIETY/WORRY:

Bergamot, Chamomile, Frankincense, Geranium, Jasmine, Lavender, Marjoram, Melissa, Neroli, Orange, Patchouli, Rose, Rosewood, Sandalwood, Vetiver, Ylang Ylang

Usage: Massage, Bath or Handkerchief/Flannel. See notes on 'Your Rescue Kit & How to Create a Blend'.

PANIC:

Benzoin, Bergamot, Frankincense, Lavender, Neroli, Rose, Ylang Ylang

Usage: Bath or Handkerchief/Flannel. See notes on 'Your Rescue Kit & How to Create a Blend'.

FEAR:

Bergamot, Chamomile, Frankincense, Geranium, Jasmine, Lavender, Marjoram, Neroli, Orange, Patchouli, Rose, Sandalwood, Vetiver, Ylang Ylang

Usage: Massage, Bath or Handkerchief/Flannel. See notes on 'Your Rescue Kit & How to Create a Blend'.

FROM YOUR 'RECOMMENDED CARRIER OILS':

GRAPE SEED
Inexpensive
Preferably for the body

BENEFITS:
Fine texture, absorbs easily into the skin, almost odourless, suitable for all skin types including sensitive, tones and purifies the skin, high fatty acid content which aids skin cell regeneration.

JOJOBA
Expensive
For the face or body

BENEFITS:
Chemically similar to human sebum, is actually a wax not an oil and therefore is excellent for protecting and nourishing the skin, has a natural SPF5 good for all skin types including sensitive.

SUNFLOWER
Inexpensive
For face or body

BENEFITS:
Absorbs quickly into the skin, contains more Vitamin E than any other carrier oil, softens the skin, good for all skin types including sensitive.

ADDITIONAL ADVICE:

FOR STRESS

- Eat more broccoli, spinach, asparagus and other dark green vegetables.

- Eat a small amount of sugary food.

- Eat complex carbohydrates (for example, oatmeal or whole grain bread) and sweet potatoes.

- Eat more oily fish (such as salmon) and turkey.

- Eat lean, grass fed beef.

- Eat some dark chocolate (70% cocoa or more).

- Eat more dairy products (such as yoghurt) (unless you have an allergy to dairy).

- Drink milk (unless you have an allergy to it).

- Chamomile tea and/or Green tea (approx 2 cups per day).

- Eat more oranges and berries (for Vitamin C and antioxidants).

FOR ANXIETY/WORRY/FEAR
As well as the list above:

- Eat more fruit, especially bananas.

- Drink Ginger tea and/or Valerian tea.

- One of the most important remedies for stress, anxiety, worry & fear would be to **relax**, and one of the best ways to do so is to practice **meditation**. Meditation will enable you to reconnect to peace and love (or God/Source/Spirit/Universe etc, depending on your personal belief) - which is the opposite of fear, and is its antidote.

- Stress comes from your **own thoughts about** the world/situations, not from the world/situations themselves. Stress is an illusion (not a tangible thing), and changing your thoughts will change your levels of stress.

- Find books to read about stress relief, including those which look at it from a more spiritual perspective and changing your thoughts (if you are interested in such things), inc. subjects such as 'living in the now/present'.

- The power of connecting to others is incredibly important, either via soothing touch, such as having a **massage**, or communicating via **talking** and getting support from other people you respect (it is important to 'let out' your worries, rather than 'bottling them up', and it is ok to cry, as this is your body's way of healing itself).

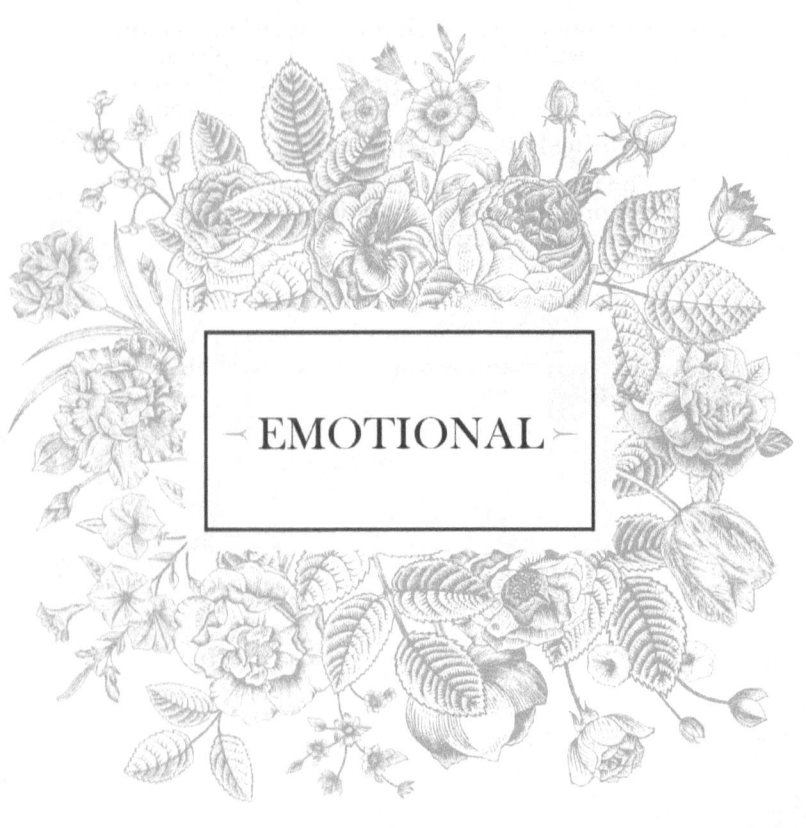

EMOTIONAL

14

BEST ESSENTIAL OILS FOR UNFORGIVENESS, ANGER & JEALOUSY

From your 'Rescue Toolkit' essential oils:

Bergamot
Chamomile
Frankincense
Geranium
Jasmine

Lavender
Orange
Rose
Neroli
Ylang Ylang

ADDITIONAL ESSENTIAL OILS:

Marjoram
Patchouli

Rosewood

ANGER/IRRITABILITY:
Bergamot, Chamomile, Geranium, Jasmine, Lavender, Neroli, Patchouli, Rosewood, Ylang Ylang

Usage: Massage, Bath or Handkerchief/Flannel. See notes on 'Your Rescue Kit & How to Create a Blend'

UNFORGIVENESS/RESENTMENT:
Chamomile, Frankincense, Geranium, Jasmine, Lavender, Rosewood, Ylang Ylang

Usage: Massage, Bath or Handkerchief/Flannel. See notes on 'Your Rescue Kit & How to Create a Blend'

BITTERNESS:
Chamomile, Frankincense, Geranium, Lavender, Marjoram, Neroli, Orange, Rose, Ylang Ylang

Usage: Massage, Bath or Handkerchief/Flannel. See notes on 'Your Rescue Kit & How to Create a Blend'

JEALOUSY:
Bergamot, Chamomile, Frankincense, Lavender, Marjoram, Orange, Rose, Ylang Ylang. Also look at the notes for 'Best Essential oils for Stress, Anxiety, Worry & Fear'

Usage: Massage, Bath or Handkerchief/Flannel. See notes on 'Your Rescue Kit & How to Create a Blend'

FROM YOUR 'RECOMMENDED CARRIER OILS':

GRAPE SEED
Inexpensive
Preferably for the body

BENEFITS:
Fine texture, absorbs easily into the skin, almost odourless, suitable for all skin types including sensitive, tones and purifies the skin, high fatty acid content which aids skin cell regeneration.

Jojoba
Expensive
For the face or body

BENEFITS:
Chemically similar to human sebum, is actually a wax not an oil and therefore is excellent for protecting and nourishing the skin, has a natural SPF5 good for all skin types including sensitive.

Sunflower
Inexpensive
For face or body

BENEFITS:
Absorbs quickly into the skin, contains more Vitamin E than any other carrier oil, softens the skin, good for all skin types including sensitive.

ADDITIONAL ADVICE:

* Anger itself is a natural, healthy emotion, and only becomes problematic when it is constant, unexpressed, unresolved or held on to long term.

* Remember that long term (constant/unexpressed/unresolved) anger/resentment/bitterness does not hurt the other person, only you. Also, it does not change the situation.

* Long term anger, unforgiveness and bitterness has the potential to manifest as physical and/or mental problems. The antidote is always forgiveness, love and peace. This doesn't mean you are condoning what the person has done to you, only that you are setting yourself free from the 'prison of bitterness'.

* Only you control what you think about, and you become what you think about. If you become an angry, bitter person this will only hurt you.

Therefore, change your thoughts to more positive ones.

- Wish peace and love for those you resent. Very difficult to do at first, but over time, this process will actually help <u>you</u> to feel more peaceful.

- Don't do things for others if you (secretly) want something in return.

- Let go of/lower your expectations of people.

- Often think about the things that you are grateful for.

- Understanding and forgiveness (towards yourself and others) are the keys for all of the 'Emotional Issues'. Learn as much as you can about this subject, and then put into practice.

15

BEST ESSENTIAL OILS
FOR
GRIEF, CHANGE & LOSS

From your 'Rescue Toolkit' essential oils:

Bergamot   Lavender
Chamomile   Neroli
Frankincense   Rose
Geranium

ADDITIONAL ESSENTIAL OILS:

Marjoram   Sandalwood

GRIEF (RESPONSE TO LOSS)/CHANGE/LOSS:
Chamomile, Frankincense, Geranium, Lavender, Neroli, Rose, Sandalwood

Usage: Massage, Bath or Handkerchief/Flannel. See notes on 'Your Rescue Kit & How to Create a Blend'
LONELINESS:

*Bergamot, Chamomile, Frankincense, Marjoram,
Rose*

Usage: Massage, Bath or Handkerchief/Flannel. See
notes on 'Your Rescue Kit & How to Create a Blend'

FROM YOUR 'RECOMMENDED CARRIER OILS':

GRAPE SEED
Inexpensive
Preferably for the body

BENEFITS:
Fine texture, absorbs easily into the skin, almost
odourless, suitable for all skin types including
sensitive, tones and purifies the skin, high fatty acid
content which aids skin cell regeneration.

JOJOBA
Expensive
For the face or body

BENEFITS:
Chemically similar to human sebum, is actually a wax
not an oil and therefore is excellent for protecting
and nourishing the skin, has a natural SPF5 good for
all skin types including sensitive.

SUNFLOWER
Inexpensive
For face or body

BENEFITS:
Absorbs quickly into the skin, contains more
Vitamin E than any other carrier oil, softens the skin,

good for all skin types including sensitive.

You might find that essential oils from the lectures on Guilt and Anger complement the 'Grief, Loss & Change' oils listed above too.

ADDITIONAL ADVICE:

FIVE STAGES OF GRIEF:

Denial:
"This can't be happening to me."

Anger:
"*Why* is this happening? Who is to blame?"

Bargaining:
"Make this not happen, and in return I will ____."

Depression:
"I'm too sad to do anything."

Acceptance:
"I'm at peace with what happened."

HELP FOR GRIEF, CHANGE, LOSS & LONELINESS:

- Get support (counsellor/therapist, family/friends, support group, your faith) and distance yourself from those who aren't compassionate towards you. Spend time with nice people.

- Express yourself/find an outlet (verbal, creative, crying etc).

- Look after yourself (nutrition, exercise, sleep).

- Remember the person you've lost (keep happy mementos which are not on constant display but that you can bring out whenever you feel the need, remember them also in your thoughts/words/deeds).

- Re-connect with things that give you peace (for example: gardening, walking, writing, voluntary work etc).

- Spend time in nature/outside.

- Don't rush your grieving process.

- Equally, don't feel guilty for moving on once you're ready. It doesn't mean you have forgotten or stopped loving the person you've lost.

This information is intended to complement medical treatment/medication, not as a replacement.

16

BEST ESSENTIAL OILS FOR LOVE, ROMANCE & SEXUALITY

From your 'Rescue Toolkit' essential oils:

Frankincense	Neroli
Geranium	Rose
Jasmine	Rosewood
Orange	Ylang Ylang

ADDITIONAL ESSENTIAL OILS:

Patchouli	Sandalwood

LOVE
Jasmine, Rose, Sandalwood, Ylang Ylang

Usage: Massage or Bath. See notes on 'Your Rescue Kit & How to Create a Blend'.

ROMANCE/PASSION
Jasmine, Orange, Patchouli, Rose, Rosewood,
Sandalwood, Ylang Ylang

Usage: Massage or Bath. See notes on 'Your Rescue
Kit & How to Create a Blend'.

SEXUALITY (INC. FEAR OF
SEXUALITY)/APHRODISIAC/INCREASE LIBIDO
Geranium, Jasmine, Patchouli, Rose, Sandalwood,
Ylang Ylang

Usage: Massage or Bath. See notes on 'Your Rescue
Kit & How to Create a Blend'.

FROM YOUR 'RECOMMENDED CARRIER OILS':

GRAPE SEED
Inexpensive
Preferably for the body

BENEFITS:
Fine texture, absorbs easily into the skin, almost
odourless, suitable for all skin types including
sensitive, tones and purifies the skin, high fatty acid
content which aids skin cell regeneration.

JOJOBA
Expensive
For the face or body

BENEFITS:
Chemically similar to human sebum, is actually a wax

not an oil and therefore is excellent for protecting and nourishing the skin, has a natural SPF5 good for all skin types including sensitive.

SUNFLOWER
Inexpensive
For face or body

BENEFITS:
Absorbs quickly into the skin, contains more Vitamin E than any other carrier oil, softens the skin, good for all skin types including sensitive.

ADDITIONAL ADVICE TO INCREASE SEX DRIVE/LIBIDO:

- Eat more vegetables & salad, such as broccoli, avocados, arugula/rocket, lettuce.
- Eat fruit such as figs, berries, watermelon, any citrus fruits.
- Eat more eggs.
- Eat more oily fish, such as salmon, mackerel, tuna.
- Try drinking Ginger Tea.
- Avoid artificial sweeteners and cakes/biscuits etc.
- Avoid high-fat products (such as high-fat dairy, crisps, junk food etc).
- Decrease coffee/caffeine intake.
- Men should avoid soy products.
- Avoid fizzy drinks.
- Decrease your intake of alcohol.

17

BEST ESSENTIAL OILS
FOR SELF ESTEEM,
GUILT & SHAME

From your 'Rescue Toolkit' essential oils:

Bergamot   Neroli
Frankincense   Rose
Jasmine   Ylang Ylang

ADDITIONAL ESSENTIAL OILS:

Sandalwood   Vetiver

SELF CONFIDENCE/ESTEEM/WORTH (INC. GUILT, SHAME)
Bergamot, Frankincense, Jasmine, Neroli, Rose, Sandalwood, Ylang Ylang

Usage: Massage, Bath or Handkerchief/Flannel. See notes on 'Your Rescue Kit & How to Create a Blend'.

INSECURITY/REJECTION:
*Bergamot, Frankincense, Jasmine, Sandalwood,
Vetiver*

Usage: Massage, Bath or Handkerchief/Flannel. See
notes on 'Your Rescue Kit & How to Create a Blend'.

FROM YOUR 'RECOMMENDED CARRIER OILS':

GRAPE SEED
*Inexpensive
Preferably for the body*

BENEFITS:
Fine texture, absorbs easily into the skin, almost
odourless, suitable for all skin types including
sensitive, tones and purifies the skin, high fatty acid
content which aids skin cell regeneration.

JOJOBA
*Expensive
For the face or body*

BENEFITS:
Chemically similar to human sebum, is actually a wax
not an oil and therefore is excellent for protecting
and nourishing the skin, has a natural SPF5 good for
all skin types including sensitive.

SUNFLOWER
*Inexpensive
For face or body*

BENEFITS:
Absorbs quickly into the skin, contains more Vitamin
E than any other carrier oil, softens the skin, good
for all skin types including sensitive.

ADDITIONAL ADVICE:

- Shame and guilt are often closely linked to
depression. Seek counselling if you believe that
these feelings have become too overwhelming
and are controlling your life.

- Learn that what you do, what you have and what
others think of you are not what define you.
Listen to cd's/read books on this subject.

- Appreciate and reward yourself.

- Learn to set personal boundaries and stop doing
things to 'people please'. Listen to cd's/read
books on this subject.

- Listen to motivational/inspirational/spiritual
cd's.

- Wear clothes that you like, and that make you
feel good.

- Take care of yourself - exercise, good posture,
good hygiene.

- Tell yourself positive affirmations, ignore
negative comments from others.

- Compliment others.

- Stop your own negative thoughts and
comparing yourself to others.

- Discontinue spending time with negative people.

- Do some voluntary work.

- Believe you can make your own decisions and that they will be good decisions. Even if it turns out you made a mistake - <u>forgive yourself</u>, and continue making decisions (learn from mistakes but don't continue to beat yourself up over them).

- Live in the present/now, not the past. There are some very good books on this subject.

- Set goals and create a plan (with simple steps to make your goals easy to achieve over time) and celebrate each step you achieve.

- Do things that you enjoy and/or are good at.

- Spend time with people you enjoy being with (family, friends etc).

- Eat healthy foods.

- Drink more water.

RECOMMENDED
SUPPLIER

I have always used a company called Aromantic, for the essential oils (and other raw ingredients) for my own 'Eden Aromatics' skin care range (www.edenaromatics.co.uk), as well as for training purposes. The oils and ingredients are of an exceptional quality, the training programmes are very thorough, the staff are friendly, knowledgeable and very helpful; and the whole company is supremely ethical. I have always found that Aromantic go above and beyond my expectations, and would therefore highly recommend them to you.

Here is a little about them:

AROMANTIC
Passionate about empowering people to make their own natural cosmetics and skin care products.

Aromantic is a unique company on the forefront of providing organic and natural ingredients, recipes, equipment and courses for make-your-own, cruelty-free and high quality cosmetics, toiletries and beauty products. They sell these ingredients in affordable quantities for small businesses, complementary therapists, market traders, home crafters and individuals.

Based in the north-east of Scotland, they stock a wide range of raw materials to make your own natural and safe creams, lotions, massage products, gels, ointments, lip balms, cleansers, face masks, spa-products, shampoos, foam baths, soaps, sun creams, and make-up & deodorants. They also stock high quality essential oils, vegetable oils, fats & waxes, natural perfumes, starter packs for beginners, books, educational material and recipe brochures and run UK-wide courses from beginners to advanced on how to make your own beauty products.

Aromantic's policy on purchasing raw materials is based on a holistic perspective, which considers the products they source and stock in relation to nature and to people. They believe that they can make a difference in the world by sourcing products and raw materials that nourish and sustain both the producers and our customers and to contribute to the demand for products that conserve our precious resources and are as environmentally friendly as possible. All of Aromantic's organic products are certified by the Organic Farmers & Growers (OF&G).

The Aromantic website gives you all the inspiration and information you may need – including details of publications and courses, as well as free articles, recipes, tips and advice on making natural products.

For more information visit
www.aromantic.co.uk
or call *01309 696 900.*

ABOUT THE AUTHOR

Faye Hurley is a fully qualified aromatherapist and beauty therapist, with sixteen years of experience; in environments ranging from top health spas and hotels, through to hospices.
She is the founder of Eden Aromatics, a luxury, artisanal skincare company, which was founded to empower women, especially those who have suffered domestic abuse.
Faye is women's wellbeing activist.

www.ingramcontent.com/pod-product-compliance
Lightning Source LLC
Chambersburg PA
CBHW021210290526
45796CB00005B/29

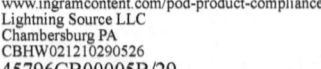